MOSAIC LIFE

MOSAIC LIFE

A Memoir in Verse

Karen Hatch-Taylor

Order this book online at www.trafford.com
or email orders@trafford.com

Most Trafford titles are also available at major online book retailers.

Printed in the United States of America.

ISBN: 978-1-4269-5167-1 (sc)
ISBN: 978-1-4269-5176-3 (e)

Trafford rev. 04/19/2011

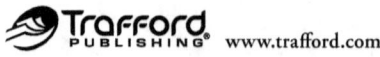 www.trafford.com

North America & international
toll-free: 1 888 232 4444 (USA & Canada)
phone: 250 383 6864 ✦ fax: 812 355 4082

For Ian.

For Ever.

Acknowledgements

I'd like to express my eternal gratitude to: my parents for their unwavering support, my siblings for their patience, Ian for true love and all the laughs, my darling children for their inspiration, and Marcia for always believing in me and for being a friend to peace and to poetry.

Additional thanks to: Holly and Charon for their lifelong friendship, Karen Richardson for those afternoons of tea and Yahtzee, Mike Rutherford and Michael Edwards for sticking with me, Dr. Apostoleris for 'getting' me, Anne and Ivan Taylor for letting me steal their son, Doctor Demento for working for so long to make people happy, Jon "Bermuda" Schwartz for going the extra mile for the fans, and lots of love and special thanks to Alfred "Weird Al" Yankovic for wanting to make people laugh and working so tirelessly to do so and for being the kind of person who brings other people together. Which brings me to: hello and thanks to Dave and Jackie and Helen and all my friends in the WOWAY, for making a community where there could have just been a crowd.

Thanks to Suzy Becker and my friend Gil L. for reminding me I'm not the only one.

But wait, there's more…my sincerest appreciation goes to Edgar Allan Poe, Emily Dickinson, Ogden Nash, Theodore Geisel, and Judith Viorst for their influence and inspiration.

And thanks again, Dad, for all the times you rescued me. And Ian...I love you. Forever.

One more thank you...to all the American servicemen and -women, and to all the veterans of the United States Armed Services...the first poem in this book is dedicated to you:

The Beach

France, 1934

"Oui, Mama" the children call
As Mama warns them not to fall
Or swim too far or step on shells
And one French mother's giving hell
To a child who didn't hover near
But hell's not here, not yet, this year
As mothers warn and scold and teach
Children at play on a sun-warmed beach

France, 1944

As the boats get near the sand
The face of every frightened man
Reflects the danger that he'll face
Here in this unfamiliar place
Where they'll dodge bullets and they'll yell
To buddies to watch out for shells
Exploding in the sandy mud
That now runs red with Allies' blood.

They've got an impossible goal to reach –
To liberate France, they must cross the beach.

USA, 2004

"Okay, Mom," the children cry
As they chase birds into the sky
The red, white, blue of the kites they fly
Are appropriate, as it's July
And last night's fireworks boomed like guns

But to the children, it was just fun.
They will not know until they're grown
That on a beach much like their own
Brave men had raced across the sand
While bullets flew at every hand
Gripping their guns, fear in their throats
(Some never made it off the boats)
As mortar shells dropped everywhere
And Allied soldiers whispered prayers.
Machine-gun fire that fell like rain
Left Normandy's beach a bloody stain.
The cause of freedom asked each man
To ship out to that foreign land
And put their very lives at stake
For freedom, and for France's sake;
Their bravery becomes the lore
Of the men who freed that foreign shore,
Sacrificing all to win the war.

But now the children play their games
Quite unaware of the many names
Engraved in stone on a shore in France
Where an army took its heroic stance.
But history someday will teach
These children the story of Omaha Beach.

Chapter 1: End of the Fantasy

Ruminations on my Divorce (In 1995, I left my lying, cheating first husband, John. He got most of the stuff, but I got our 5-year-old daughter, Angelina, so I figure I was the lucky one.)

This one's pretty self-explanatory. This is for my *former* friend Tracy:

The Other Woman

You'll always be the "other woman," no matter what you do.
You'll always be his mistress, even if he marries you.
What will your friends all think about your happy married life
When they find out you dated him while he still had a wife?
And late at night, you'll look at him and wonder, "is he true?"
He cheated on his first "true love," of course he'll cheat on *you*!
What makes you think that *you* inspire a faithfulness in men
Who've cheated on their other women? He *will* cheat again!
And when he does, at least you'll know that justice has been served.
The pain you'll feel when it's *your* turn will be what you deserve.

More...

1996
It's just before midnight
And I can't sleep
You should've told me you were evil
Just a lying, cheating creep

I need to get a life, but some other day
I never meant for things to stay this way.
Some day I'll rise and shine to greet the dawn
For now, it's just another night with the TV on.

Divorced

I've got my own place with a front door that locks
And a drawer in my bureau that's only for socks
I've got my own silverware, cups, bowls, and plates
And I've still got the big quilt he said that he hates
I've got all the photos from happier days
And I feel like a person in so many ways
But there's still a big hole in my shiny new life –
What am I now that I'm not somebody's wife?
Am I somebody else? Was I someone before?
Will I just lock myself behind my new front door?
Will anyone call me? Will I be all right?
And why am I lonely and restless all night?
It feels like I'm waiting for something to be
As if, after all of this time, there's no me.
There once was a man that I gave myself to
Now that he isn't here, I don't know what to do
I know that it's true that I have to keep going
I just didn't realize my pain would be showing
I feel like I'm wounded; my sorrow's so deep
That it haunts me all day, and then when I'm asleep
I dream of the past as if we're all still there
Then I wake up confused, and it's just so unfair.
Is he suffering, too? And should I even care?
I just feel so awful. It's just so unfair.

To a Friend, On Her Divorce

I know that you've gone into hiding --
I divorced once, so I've been there, too.
Your life right now isn't exciting;
You just do the things you have to do.

You're managing all of your "mom" stuff
And working to hold back your tears.
Right now, the going is slow, and tough;
This healing will likely take years.

But this is a note to remind you
Whenever you're at your wit's end:
Get word to me, I'll come and find you
When you're ready to talk to a friend.

I loved him right
He did me wrong
- -End of story
No more love songs

...or so I feared then...

5

Chapter 2: So Far Away

In 1996, I met an Australian writer named Ian Taylor online in the "Weird Al" Yankovic newsgroup. We were e-mail pen pals for nearly two years, during which time I read the manuscript of his first novel* and I completely fell in love with the book, the characters..and the author. I decided we were meant for each other. These poems are from that period.

* (The hilarious comedy sci-fi novel *Spindle*, pub. 2005.)

Confession

My far-off friend writes letters; they are funny, warm, and
long.
He writes me little poems; they're like pieces of a song.
I cherish every word he writes, but I don't tell him so.
(I find it hard, though, to believe that he still doesn't know.)
A dozen times or more I'll read a letter that he wrote.
I look for hidden meanings in his simplest friendly note.
And if I don't find any, I assume he's trying to hide
The same feelings I am hiding, that I keep so deep inside.
It may just be he's very sweet and has a charming style…
But when he sends me poetry, imagine how I smile!
Someday I'll get my courage up, and then what I will do
Is write my friend a note that says, "My heart belongs to you."

For My Friend

I'm sorry if what I feel for you is love
I didn't mean it to be
I know it's not what you want, but
I didn't know what you did want from me
And so I hoped that it was this, oh!
How I wanted it to be true!
But the strength of my feelings pushed you
Away, even as I felt so close to you.

Please come back.
I can't not love you, but I can pretend
That I don't always dream of you
That all you are to me is a friend.

Edge of the Sidewalk

As a child, I walked the edge of the sidewalk
Always the edge –
It's more exciting when you might fall.

As I talk to you, I can almost feel
My tiny little sneakers
Poised precariously on the brink of the concrete.

If I push too hard, I lose –
You'll know how I feel about you, and all will be lost.
Into the gutter I'll go with my tiny dreams.

But I am feeling reckless.
I think perhaps I'll lean too far
Just to see if you catch me –
All it would take are the words
"I don't want us to just be friends."

I teeter on the edge of the sidewalk
Planning, fearing, hesitating.
And when I see the way you smile at me,
Glorious falling feeling.

claws

It was like a kitten spilled from a paper bag
At first, so small, with tiny eyes and voice
On shaky legs it stood and called to me
And answer?…well, I felt I had no choice

It grew, then, like a playful kitten will
And pounced upon me every chance it got
Unleashed, untamed, it always followed me
Knew places in my heart that I did not
It, catlike, slunk so often past my mind
As if I were a mouse it soon would catch
Began to seem a little like a threat
And I began to feel I'd met my match

At last I'm overpowered by this thing
This hunger, deep desire and love for you
That holds me in its claws, a prisoner
Just like a cotton mouse a cat would chew.

And caught inside your paws and claws and teeth
As if this was the way we always were
The captured prey to the hunter does submit
And as you kiss me, I begin to purr.

(That was wishful thinking. Ian had no idea how I felt about him. But I invited him to come to America, and he was considering the possibility. *I* was considering a *number* of possibilities.)

Two Poets

Two poets half a world apart
Began a game of Share Your Heart
And laughing, each would write a verse
And humbly claim that theirs was worse
They molded words as if of clay
And language was to them just play
And thus it was for long a time
Two poets shared each other's rhyme
Like gifts exchanged, their lyrics sweet
Began to speak of when they'd meet
And cross the great ten thousand miles
To bring each other words and smiles

Two poets half a world apart
Each soothed the other's anguished heart
And filled each other's nights and days
With metaphors and lavish praise
A subtle joke, a weary sigh,
Some light sweet verse and a battle cry
Two poets wrote, would joke and flirt
To quell the darkness, ease the hurt
But always swear they'd someday meet
And write their poem soft and sweet

Two poets half a world apart
Played a game of Share Your Heart
And words would ring like distant bells
Across the great wide ocean swells
Where, when it's darkness on one side
The sunrise greets the other tide
Upon this planet cloudy blue
Two poets work on something new
I know this vision to be true
For one is me, the other you.

Chapter 3: Got 'im!

(Ian came to visit. We fell in love and got engaged. Six months later, in 1998, we were married in Australia, then settled in my home state of Massachusetts. When we found we were expecting a baby girl, Elise, in 1999, I wrote this for Angelina, who was then ten.)

Once There Were Two

I know you remember the time when it was just you and me.

Now you have a new dad
And soon the new baby
And I know that sometimes it seems like it's happening too fast.
Becoming a big family.
It's not just you and me anymore.

But I want you to know
That I'll never forget the times
When you were the only raft in my ocean of loneliness,
The only bright star in my dark sky.

You helped me, and I helped you, and together
We were not just a mother and child
But a whole family by ourselves.

Those times will never disappear from my memory
And I want you to know
That no matter how many people there are to love in my life,
I will never love you any less.
Only more, because when I am loved and happy,
I have more love to give.

Watching you grow,
Helping you become the wonderful woman that you are,
Has been my honor, and it's been fun, too.
Now, we have others to share our fun with, and to love.
But always remember this:
Nothing will ever change how very much I love you. --Mom

Chapter 4: Turn of the Century

Wow. The year 2000. All my life, I'd expected it to be a wondrous future time. Instead, it was a time of Y2K panic and a fascist overthrow of America by Bush/Cheney and their evil advisor, Karl Rove. I found it all very stressful, and on top of that, I had a one-year-old and Angelina was going through her "sullen teen" stage.

TO MY TEEN (For Angelina, 2002)

I think you revel in your misery
Can't wait to see the person you'll turn out to be
And I know it's your time to grow away from me.

I know you don't realize how much I have done for you.
When you get out on your own I don't know what you'll do
But I do know this: I love you and I'm so proud of you.

--Mom

(Thank goodness we got out of that phase more or less unscathed.)

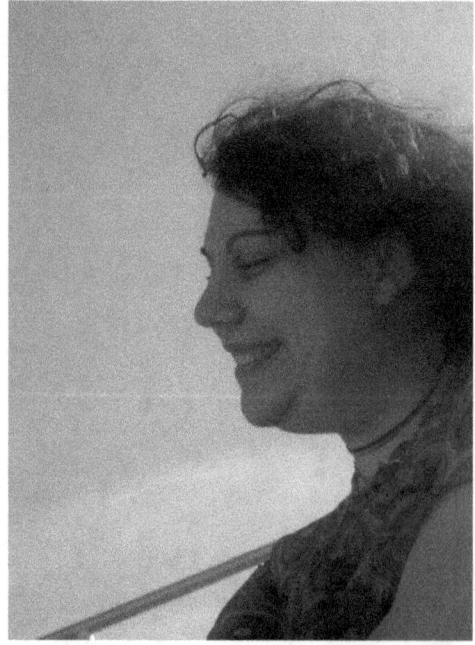

Angelina at 21

SIX YEARS ON (To Ian on Our 6th Wedding Anniversary, 2003)

Compared to our parents, it's not very long
But after six years of marriage, we know we're not wrong
You're still the best thing that ever happened to me
Six years on

We look at our children and we swell with pride
We both know that at times it's been one scary ride
But here we are now and we're both satisfied
Six years on

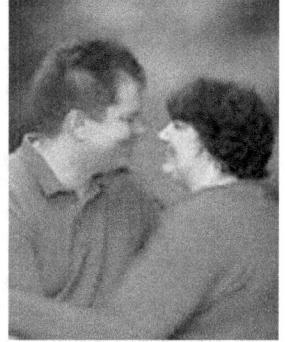

Six years without ever a thought of divorce
You're still my knight on a big white horse
You're still my hero, and my partner of course
Six years on

Ian and Karen

After six years of the honor of being your wife
Even though I laugh when you eat pancakes with a knife
I think we both know that we're in this for life
And that's fine
'Cause I'm glad you're mine

You truly are the man of my dreams
The kind who'd surprise me with a box of Krispy Kremes
Just for fun
Babe, you're the one
Six years on...and forever

(Yes, we sure thought 2003 was our year. We'd been married six years and were still in love, Angelina and Elise were healthy, and we'd found out we were expecting a son. But our plans were interrupted when doctors found a massive brain tumor in my right temporal lobe. They did a C-section to remove our son, Bennett, and then I had brain surgery a week later. Amazingly, Ben was unaffected by his early birth and has enjoyed near-perfect health. The brain surgery left me disabled, forgetful, and depressed, but I had to admit that I am lucky to be alive. And what does not kill me...inspires me!

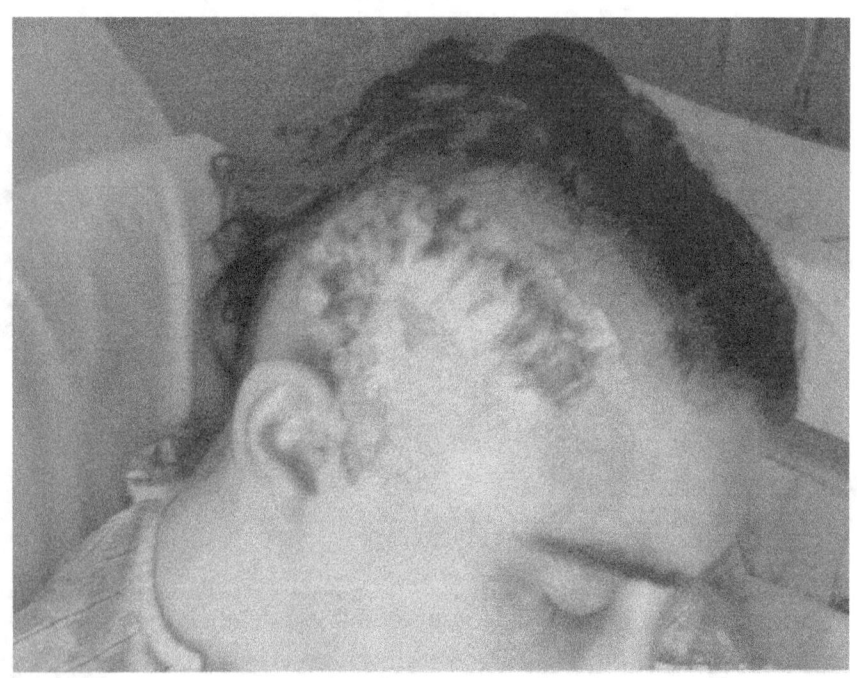
Karen after her brain surgery, May 2003

Chapter 5: Balance

Brain Surgery

The worst part's not the surgery
The worst part's not the scar
The worst part is not knowing
If it has altered who you are.

My friends say I'll get better
But they don't understand
What it's like to feel confused this way
And I can't use my left hand!
My balance is really bad now
So don't ask me to walk down stairs
And my hair grew back pretty fast somehow
(I wish my brain had, too, but hey, life's not fair.)
They tell me the surgery saved my life
So to wish it hadn't happened would be dumb
And I can still be a mother, still be a wife
So I guess I'm okay with who I've become

I touch my temple and feel the titanium plate
I know it's a miracle I'm doing great
I'm coming to terms with the fear and pain
My friend, my enemy, my self – my brain.

Brain Surgery (2)

They all said, "we're amazed at how you're coping,
And we're hoping that you get well very soon."
And their good wishes were apparent in reminders --
Every card, bouquet of flowers, and balloon.
But the cards said "Get Well *Soon*," not *"Eventually,"*
And I thought perhaps with wishes such as those
The healing might proceed rather speedily.
But still disabled, I watched the death of every rose.

The flowers are all dead now, the cards all put away
And no one likes to talk about that time
The only proof I have it ever happened
Is that my therapy is still an uphill climb.

And the plate screwed to my skull that I can feel under my skin—
When I think about what happened, I still can barely take it in.

In 2003, we also found out that our beautiful little girl, Elise, has Asperger Syndrome, a form of autism. It was devastating news. I struggle daily to understand her and help her learn to live in a world she can't comprehend.

Elise enjoys Japanese culture, so I wrote about her in haikus:

Elise haiku

Elise is a girl
She has Asperger Syndrome
And she's a genius.

Beautiful daughter;
Horrible daily meltdowns.
Our love can't stop them.

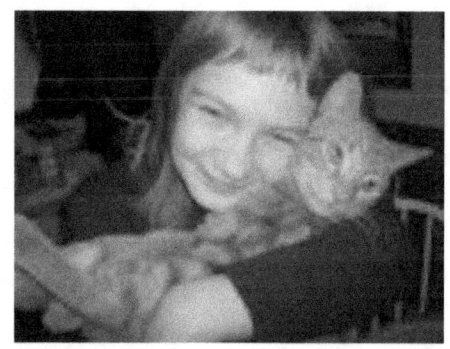

Elise with her best friend, our cat Crazy Cat.

Unusual girl,
Your struggles make me so sad.
How can I help you?

- love always, Mom.

As if a brain tumor weren't devastating enough, in 2005, I was diagnosed with cancer (Hodgkin's Lymphoma) and endured a grueling regimen of chemo/radiation. I was terrified, but also inspired. I hope these poems will be a comfort to others dealing with cancer.

"Big C" 1

Was it the stuff that I put in my coffee?
Was it the toppings on my pizza pie?
What could have made me of all people get cancer?
I can't believe there's a chance I could die!
It's all so unfair and I need to know why.
What if…what if…oh no! OH MY!!
What if it's random, and there *isn't* a why?
The universe fires a random shot
And this time it seems I'm the one that it got.
I don't smoke, I don't drink, I don't steal, I don't lie
But I have cancer, and it seems there's no answer to "why?"
I'm the one in my family who didn't drink or smoke –
So, what, is my diagnosis some odd cosmic joke?

"Big C" 2

Listen, Cancer, damn nuisance they call the "Big C" –
You may be tough, but I think you've met your match in me.
I have so much to live for, so much living to do!
And I won't give that up for a freak thing like you.
My doctors and I have a plan that can win
So don't think for a second that I might give in.
The chemo does make me feel sick, but I'll live –
I can certainly beat any resistance you give.
So you think you're so tough 'cause they call you "Big C?"
Well, I'm tougher than you; you know what they call *me*?

S U R V I V O R !!

When I had cancer, my then-four-year-old son developed an alter ego: Happy Man, a superhero who gave people hugs "to make them feel better." You could say it was just a young child's way of dealing with a parent's serious illness, but I would swear that those hugs from Happy Man are the reason I beat the cancer. (That and the chemo. But hugs make me happy, and chemo makes me puke my guts out.)

About My Son

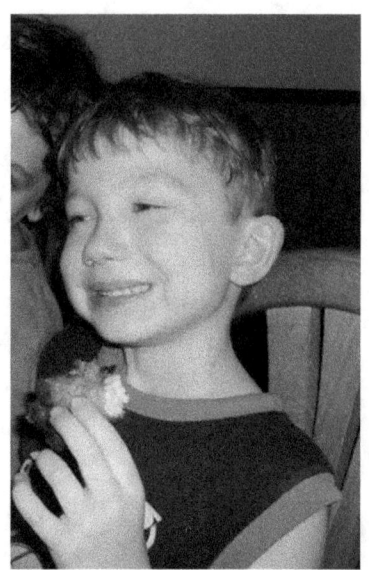

Of my three kids, the youngest one
Is my boy Bennett, my only son.
He's sweet and smart and loves to hug
And play with Legos on the rug.
I taught him to read when he was four.
He's just too easy to adore,
My darling little honeybun.
No one loves me like my son.
I love to feel him kiss my cheek.
When he plays alone, I like to peek.
I love to watch him having fun.
'Cause no one loves me like my son.

Bennett at 7

Three kids, autism, cancer, disabilities…it got to feel like too much sometimes. I wrote this next poem to explain why I felt so stressed out at that point:

Too Much on my Plate

Three children really isn't so many
I feel awful for people who can't have any.
The kids do cause me stress, but I know
It's a lot of work to care for them, that is so,
With all the feeding and bathing and changing and dressing
But even when I'm changing diapers, I always know
That every little baby is a blessing.

I always wanted to own my own house
With a dryer and a washing machine
Now I have one, so okay, I guess I won't grouse,
But why can't I ever get the whole place clean?!?
Between the house and the kids and pleasing my mate,
It's clear I've just got too much on my plate.

I feel I should be able to single-handedly do this stuff –
Pay the bills (there's no money), keep the house clean, and spend time
with each kid
It means a to-do list with a million items (pretty rough)
But, hey, it isn't any more than my *own* mom did.

Women's magazines advise me how to keep things organized,
And cook fine meals and rich desserts, all while losing twenty pounds!
How to knit a lovely sweater (except, I'm oversized),
And of course in every issue, advice abounds
About the ways to make kids listen to you
So they can all do well in school and turn out great
As if anyone could help my poor children through this
When their mother has just got too much on her plate.

But if I don't do well at how I raise them
Their whole lives will be ruined; the stakes are high.
I have to remember not to yell, but to praise them
But right now the little one's spitting yogurt in my eye.
And I'm holding a stack of somebody's school papers from today,
And that glass is about to slide off of that shelf,
And the magazine suggests that after I make a fresh parmesan soufflé,
I should "take a little time out for myself."
When my husband comes home from work at last to find me in this state,
And asks why I'm crying, I say, "I've just got too much on my plate."

Don't try to be a Superwoman, the magazines insist,
But…redecorate, keep a budget, always cook great meals.
Exercise 'til both your thighs are thinner than your wrist,
Raise perfect children, and still negotiate great deals.
(The one thing I never see in their table of contents
Is any indication they understand how a woman feels.)

Before last year, there wasn't anything wrong with the way we live.
I was a great mom, I had things in check, I was my husband's happy lover
Since they found my brain tumor, I just don't seem to have any more to give.
I couldn't have ever imagined that it takes this long to recover.
They did get most of the tumor out; it seems I will survive.
But can my family ever forgive me for what this has done to all our lives?

When someone suggests that I really should do something about my weight,
And I realize I had an appointment and I'm now two hours late,
And I'll never pay off my mortgage barring some lucrative twist of fate,
I think the whole family could end up in a nuthouse at this rate.

When I run into friends they always say,
"I see you're doing great."
There's no way to explain to them
I've just got too much on my plate.

Chapter 6: Politics

(I was inspired by events of the early 2000s to write poetry that's much more political than my earlier work. If anything I've written conflicts with anyone's personal politics, they should feel free to ignore it.)

Footage

I see the old newsreel footage
Grainy black and white footage of blacks and whites
People marching, Alabama cities
Children trying to get to their school.

It's not like that now, I reason.
The marching made a difference.
But as I watch the footage, I see myself
Marching for the civil rights of my fellow man.
And I promise myself that if I'd been born 50 years earlier, I'd have marched, too,
even though I'm white.
Because I believe in equal rights for all.

I turn on the evening news
And see the footage, in full color.
People marching, in Boston and San Francisco.
People trying to get legally wed.

It will happen, I reason.
The marching will carry the message.
And as I watch the footage, I ask myself
"Don't I care about the rights of my fellow man?"
And I promise myself that tomorrow, I will march too,
Even though I'm straight.
Because I believe in equal rights for all.

And because tomorrow it could be one of my friends or one of my kids
Who just wants to declare their eternal love for another person.
And no law is going to stop them, not as long as I have the strength to march.
Why do you think they call it "footage?"

July 2004, War with Iraq

I don't believe what they told me about the war
I don't think anyone knew what we were fighting for
I believe in my nation – ♥America! – and love it from shore to
shore
But I don't believe what they told me
Told me about this war

I know it can be said, in general, that war is very bad
And when I hear that someone died from my own state, I get
so mad
Because I know his family must be so sad to lose someone they
adore
And it's worse when we can't even believe what they tell us
Tell us about this war

I was in the crowd on the Fourth, watching fireworks, calling
for more
Full of patriotism, feeling American right to the core
But I just don't trust our President*; I wish we could show him
the door
I'm afraid and I think he's lying to all of us
Lying about this war

---

*Then-Acting President (and I **do** mean *acting*) GW Bush

Nine Hundred Families

2004 is a scary time
Sometimes I lie awake at night
And I can see the faces of crying moms
Siblings and little kids, husbands and wives
Who've lost someone they truly need
Because of something our president* did
Out of anger and oil greed

He can say now he ousted a bad bad man
But I remember that when the war began
He claimed we were going for our own defense
But now he blames incorrect documents
Now over nine hundred families mourn and weep
I see their faces when I try to sleep

He swore to us it was time for war
But what did he really destroy those families for?
I think our president's* a bad bad man
And I think the world is devising a plan
To knock down that bully they find so scary
Save America – in November, vote for John Kerry!

(We did! But Senator Kerry became the second duly-elected president who couldn't serve his term because GW Bush was squatting in the White House. Strange days indeed.)

*Then-Acting President (and I **do** mean *acting*) GW Bush

Dénouement

In 2007, I was done with cancer (in remission), what's left of my brain tumor seemed to be inactive, and the kids were healthy. Angelina graduated high school and left for college. Elise and Bennett played and fought like all siblings, and I dared hope my woes were over. It was around this time that I was diagnosed with Type 2 Diabetes. It'll be a lifelong struggle, but if anyone can beat it, I can.

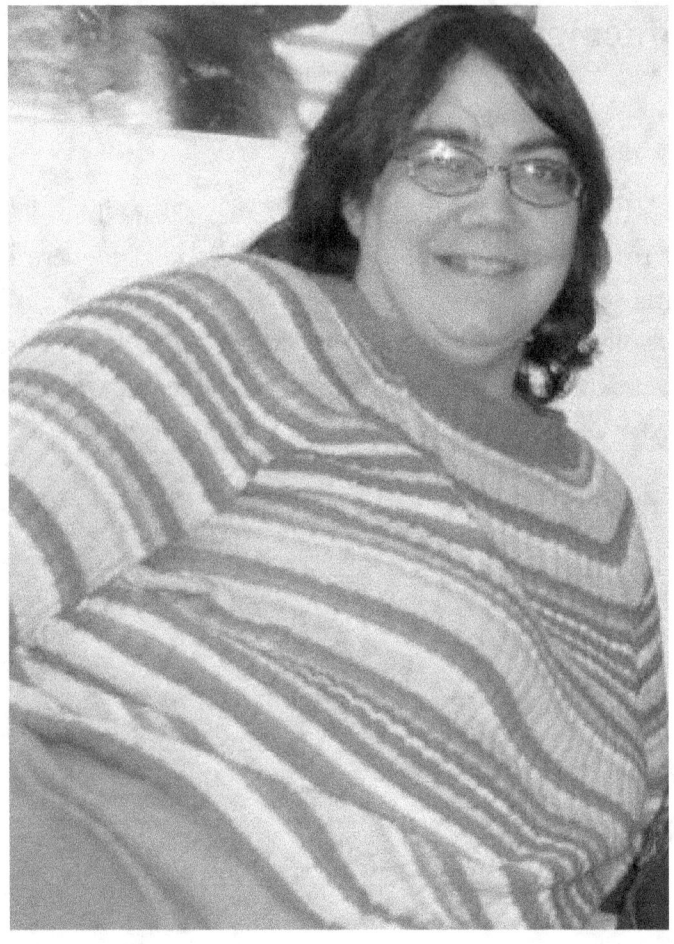

Karen Hatch Taylor is a brain-tumor survivor and full-time mom who grew up in Central Massachusetts and lives there with her husband, Australian comedy writer Ian Taylor (author of *Spindle*), and their three children.

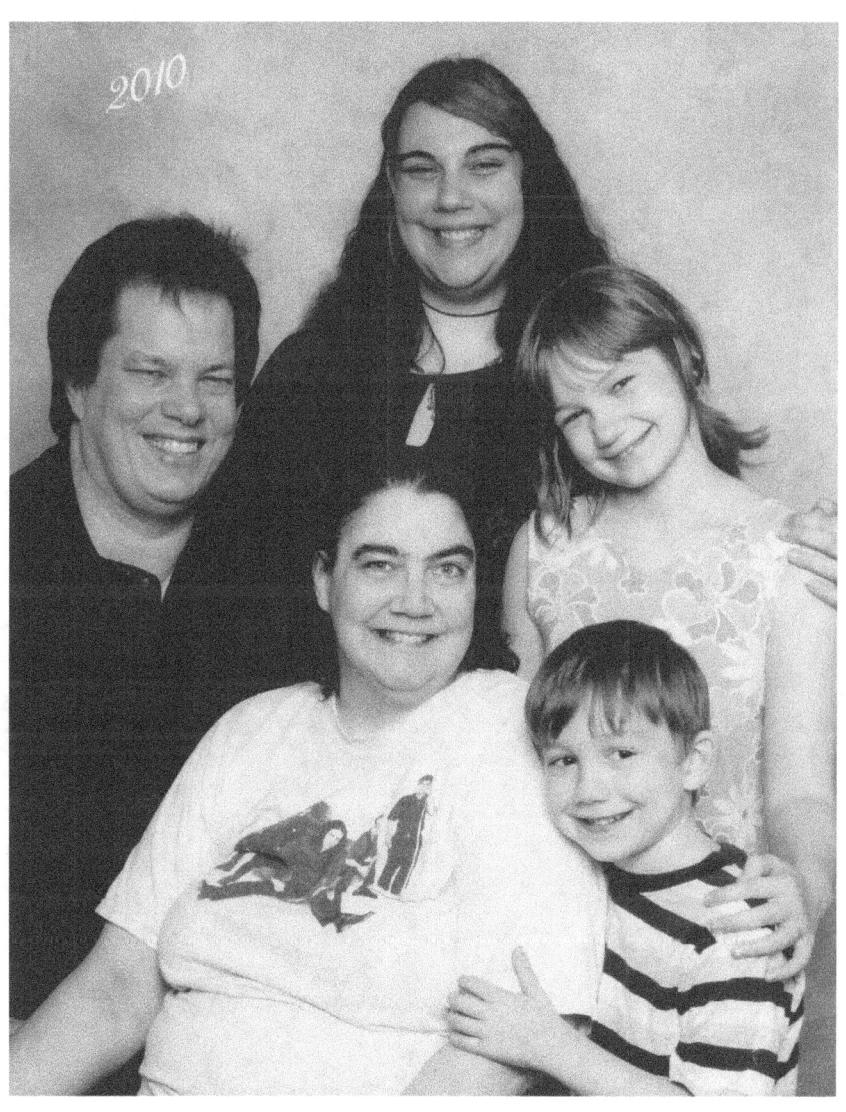

Karen and her family in September 2010.

www.ingramcontent.com/pod-product-compliance
Lightning Source LLC
Chambersburg PA
CBHW070842310526
45793CB00011B/501